CIRRHOSIS COOKBOOK

Breakfast, Main Course, Dessert and Snacks Recipes for Cirrhosis

TABLE OF CONTENTS

BREAKFAST 6

"GOOD MORNING" BROWNIES 6

BANANA OATMEAL 8

MORNING SMOOTHIE 9

MORNING CUSTARD 10

CHINESE OMELET 11

BLUEBERRIES OATMEAL 12

CHIA PUDDING 13

BREAKFAST CASSEROLE 14

BLUEBERRY BALLS 16

BREAKFAST COOKIES 17

LUNCH 20

POTATO SALAD 20

CARROT SALAD 22

MOROCCAN SALAD 23

AVOCADO CHICKEN SALAD 25

CUCUMBER SALAD 27

VEGETABLE SOUP 29

PARSNIP SOUP 31

ASPARAGUS SOUP 33

ONION SOUP 35

ZUCCHINI SOUP 37

TURKEY BURGERS 39

ROASTED SALMON 41

LUNCH NOODLES 42

CAULIFLOWER WINGS	43
LETTUCE CHICKEN WRAPS	45
DINNER	**48**
EASY OYSTERS	48
DINER CHILI	50
GINGER SALMON	52
PORK TACOS	53
VEGETABLE STEW	55
STUFFED SWEET POTATOES	56
CHICKEN AND RICE	58
LIVER AND MASHED VEGETABLES	59
LEMON CHICKEN	61
CLASSIC LIVER AND ONION	63
DINNER BURGERS	64
DINNER NACHOS	66
STUFFED PEPPERS	68
PORK TACOS	70
FISH TACOS	72
SMOOTHIES	**75**
GREEN SMOOTHIE	75
CLEANSE SMOOTHIE	76
DETOX SMOOTHIE	77
ZUCCHINI AND AVOCADO SMOOTHIE	78
TURMERIC SMOOTHIE	79
PUMPKIN SPICE SMOOTHIE	80
CARROT SMOOTHIE	81

EASY SMOOTHIE	82
BEET SMOOTHIE	83
ORANGE SMOOTHIE	84
DESSERTS	**86**
CHIA PUDDING	86
CHOCOLATE FUDGE PIE	87
PEACH PARFAIT	88
BANANA PUDDING	90
EASY BLONDIES	92
DATE BALLS	94
NUTELLA	95
APPLE CRUMBLE	96
SWEET POTATO CUSTARD	98
CACAO TRUFFLES	99

Copyright 2019 by Noah Jerris - All rights reserved.

This document is geared towards providing exact and reliable information in regards to the topic and issue covered. The publication is sold with the idea that the publisher is not required to render accounting, officially permitted, or otherwise, qualified services. If advice is necessary, legal or professional, a practiced individual in the profession should be ordered.

- From a Declaration of Principles which was accepted and approved equally by a Committee of the American Bar Association and a Committee of Publishers and Associations.

In no way is it legal to reproduce, duplicate, or transmit any part of this document in either electronic means or in printed format. Recording of this publication is strictly prohibited and any storage of this document is not allowed unless with written permission from the publisher. All rights reserved.

The information provided herein is stated to be truthful and consistent, in that any liability, in terms of inattention or otherwise, by any usage or abuse of any policies, processes, or directions contained within is the solitary and utter responsibility of the recipient reader. Under no circumstances will any legal responsibility or blame be held against the publisher for any reparation, damages, or monetary loss due to the information herein, either directly or indirectly.

Respective authors own all copyrights not held by the publisher.

The information herein is offered for informational purposes solely, and is universal as so. The presentation of the information is without contract or any type of guarantee assurance.

The trademarks that are used are without any consent, and the publication of the trademark is without permission or backing by the trademark owner. All trademarks and brands within this book are for clarifying purposes only and are the owned by the owners themselves, not affiliated with this document.

Introduction

Cirrhosis recipes for personal enjoyment but also for family enjoyment. You will love them for sure for how easy it is to prepare them.

BREAKFAST

"GOOD MORNING" BROWNIES

Serves: **10**

Prep Time: **5** Minutes

Cook Time: **15** Minutes

Total Time: **20** Minutes

INGREDIENTS

- 15 oz black beans
- 1/3 cup oats
- 1/3 tsp salt
- 1 ½ tbs sugar
- ½ cup maple syrup
- 2 ½ tbs cocoa powder
- 3 tbs vanilla
- 1 tsp baking powder
- 1 cup chocolate chips
- 1/3 cup coconut oil

DIRECTIONS

1. **Preheat the oven to 375F**

2. Blend all ingredients together except chocolate chips
3. Fold in the chocolate chips and pour the batter into a greased pan
4. Cook for at least 15 minutes
5. Allow to cool then cut and serve

BANANA OATMEAL

Serves: **4**

Prep Time: **10** Minutes

Cook Time: **8** Hours

Total Time: **8** Hours

INGREDIENTS

- 1 cup oats
- 1/3 tsp salt
- 3 tbs almond butter
- 3 cups water
- 2 bananas
- 2 tbs honey
- 1 ½ cups milk

DIRECTIONS

1. Mix water, milk, salt and oats and place in a slow cooker
2. Cook covered for about 8 hours
3. Place into bowls, add almond butter and honey and top with banana slices
4. Serve

MORNING SMOOTHIE

Serves: 1
Prep Time: 2 Minutes
Cook Time: 3 Minutes
Total Time: 5 Minutes

INGREDIENTS

- ½ cup raspberries
- 1/3 cup red beets
- 2 tbs nut butter
- 1 tsp flax oil
- 1 ½ cup coconut water
- 1/3 banana
- 1 cup yogurt
- ½ cup kale
- ½ cup blueberries

DIRECTIONS

1. Blend all ingredients together
2. Serve immediately

MORNING CUSTARD

Serves: 2

Prep Time: **10** Minutes

Cook Time: **10** Minutes

Total Time: **20** Minutes

INGREDIENTS

- 5 tbs chia seeds
- 1 cup coconut milk
- 3 tbs honey
- 1/3 tsp cinnamon
- 1 tsp vanilla
- 1 cup yogurt
- 1/3 tsp sumac
- 1/3 cup orange juice

DIRECTIONS

1. Mix sumac and chia seeds with cinnamon in a blender
2. Add milk, orange juice, yogurt, honey and vanilla
3. Pulse a little more
4. Allow to rest in the fridge for at least an hour

CHINESE OMELET

Serves: *1*

Prep Time: *5* Minutes

Cook Time: *5* Minutes

Total Time: *10* Minutes

INGREDIENTS

- 2 eggs
- 1/3 cup tomato
- 1/3 cup kale
- 1/3 cup green onion
- 1 ½ tbs sour cream
- 2 tsp garlic

DIRECTIONS

1. Whisk the eggs and sour cream together until light
2. Saute the chopped vegetables for about 3 minutes
3. Pour in the eggs and cook until done
4. Serve immediately

BLUEBERRIES OATMEAL

Serves: **2**

Prep Time: **10** Minutes

Cook Time: **8** Hours

Total Time: **8** Hours

INGREDIENTS

- 1/3 cup oats
- 1/3 cup blueberries
- 2 tbs maple syrup
- 1/3 cup coconut milk
- ½ tsp vanilla
- 1 banana
- 1 ½ tsp chia seeds

DIRECTIONS

1. Mix the oats and chia seeds together
2. Pour in the milk and top with blueberries and sliced banana
3. Refrigerate for at least 8 hours
4. Stir in the maple syrup and serve

CHIA PUDDING

Serves: 2
Prep Time: 5 Minutes
Cook Time: 10 Minutes
Total Time: 15 Minutes

INGREDIENTS

- 5 tbs chia seeds
- 1 ½ tbs vanilla
- 2 tbs maple syrup
- 2 ½ cup almond milk
- 1 ½ cup strawberries
- 1 beet

DIRECTIONS

1. Blend together the milk, strawberries, chopped beet, maple syrup, and vanilla
2. Pour into a cup and ad the chia
3. Stir every 5 minutes for 15 minutes
4. Refrigerate overnight
5. Serve topped with fruits

BREAKFAST CASSEROLE

Serves: **4**
Prep Time: **10** Minutes
Cook Time: **35** Minutes
Total Time: **45** Minutes

INGREDIENTS

- 7 oz asparagus
- 3 tbs parsley
- 1 cup broccoli
- 1 zucchini
- 3 tbs oil
- 5 eggs
- Salt
- Pepper

DIRECTIONS

1. Cook the diced zucchini, asparagus and broccoli florets in heated oil for about 5 minutes
2. Season with salt and pepper and remove from heat
3. Whisk the eggs and season then add the parsley

4. Place the vegetables in a greased pan then pour the eggs over
5. Bake in the preheated oven for about 35 minutes at 350F
6. Serve warm

BLUEBERRY BALLS

Serves: **12**

Prep Time: **5** Minutes

Cook Time: **30** Minutes

Total Time: **35** Minutes

INGREDIENTS

- 2 cups oats
- 1 cup blueberries
- 1/3 cup honey
- 1 tsp cinnamon
- 1 ½ tsp vanilla
- 1/3 cup almond butter

DIRECTIONS

1. Mix the honey, vanilla, oats, almond butter, and cinnamon together
2. Fold in the blueberries
3. Refrigerate for at least 30 minutes
4. Form balls from the dough and serve

BREAKFAST COOKIES

Serves: **15**

Prep Time: **10** Minutes

Cook Time: **40** Minutes

Total Time: **50** Minutes

INGREDIENTS

- 1 cup oats
- 2 tsp vanilla
- 1/3 cup honey
- ¼ tsp salt
- 2 ½ tbs coconut oil
- 1 egg
- 1 cup apple
- 1 cup flour
- 2 tsp baking powder
- 2 tsp cinnamon

DIRECTIONS

1. Mix the flour, oats, cinnamon, baking powder, and salt together
2. Mix the coconut butter, egg and vanilla well, then add the honey
3. Mix the wet and dry ingredients together then add the diced apple
4. Refrigerate for at least 30 minutes
5. Divide the dough into 15 scoops on a lined baking sheet
6. Bake in the preheated oven for about 15 minutes at 320F
7. Allow to cool the serve

LUNCH

POTATO SALAD

Serves: 2

Prep Time: 5   Minutes

Cook Time: 10   Minutes

Total Time: 15   Minutes

INGREDIENTS

- 5 potatoes
- 1 tsp cumin seeds
- 1/3 cup oil
- 2 tsp mustard
- 1 red onion
- 2 cloves garlic
- 1/3 cup lemon juice
- 1 tsp sea salt

DIRECTIONS

1. Steam the potatoes until tender
2. Mix mustard, turmeric powder, lemon juice, cumin seeds, and salt

3. Place the potatoes in a bowl and pour the lemon mixture over
4. Add the chopped onion and minced garlic over
5. Stir to coat and refrigerate covered
6. Add oil and stir before serving

CARROT SALAD

Serves: 2
Prep Time: 5 Minutes
Cook Time: 5 Minutes
Total Time: 10 Minutes

INGREDIENTS

- 1 ½ tbs lemon juice
- 1/3 tsp salt
- ¼ tsp black pepper
- 2 tbs olive oil
- 1/3 lb carrots
- 1 tsp mustard

DIRECTIONS

1. Mix mustard, lemon juice and oil together
2. Peel and shred the carrots in a bowl
3. Stir in the dressing and season with salt and pepper
4. Mix well and allow to chill for at least 30 minutes
5. Serve

MOROCCAN SALAD

Serves: 2

Prep Time: 5 Minutes

Cook Time: 5 Minutes

Total Time: 10 Minutes

INGREDIENTS

- 2 tbs lemon juice
- 1 tsp cumin
- 1 tsp paprika
- 3 tbs olive oil
- 2 cloves garlic
- 5 carrots
- Salt
- Pepper

DIRECTIONS

1. Peel and slice the carrots
2. Add the carrots in boiled water and simmer for at least 5 minutes
3. Drain and rinse the carrots under cold water
4. Add in a bowl

5. Mix the lemon juice, garlic, cumin, paprika, and olive oil together
6. Pour the mixture over the carrots and toss then season with salt and pepper
7. Serve immediately

AVOCADO CHICKEN SALAD

Serves: 2
Prep Time: 5 Minutes
Cook Time: 5 Minutes
Total Time: 10 Minutes

INGREDIENTS

- 3 tsp lime juice
- 3 tbs cilantro
- 1 chicken breast
- 1 avocado
- 1/3 cup onion
- 1 apple
- 1 cup celery
- Salt
- Pepper
- Olive oil

DIRECTIONS

1. Dice the chicken breast
2. Season with salt and pepper and cook into a greased skillet until golden

3. Dice the vegetables and place over the chicken in a bowl
4. Mash the avocado and sprinkle in the cilantro
5. Season with salt and pepper and add lime juice
6. Serve drizzled with olive oil

CUCUMBER SALAD

Serves: *8*

Prep Time: *5* Minutes

Cook Time: *5* Minutes

Total Time: *10* Minutes

INGREDIENTS

- 2 cucumbers
- ½ cup vinegar
- 2 tsp sugar
- 1/3 cup water
- 2 tbs sour cream
- ½ tbs salt
- 1 ½ tsp paprika
- ½ onion

DIRECTIONS

1. Peel and slice the cucumbers
2. Place the cucumbers on a baking sheet and sprinkle with salt
3. Allow to chill for about 30 minutes then squeeze out the excess water

4. Place the onion slices in a bowl and add the drained cucumbers over
5. Add water, sugar, vinegar and paprika
6. Allow to marinate for at least 2 hours
7. Serve

VEGETABLE SOUP

Serves: **8**

Prep Time: **10** Minutes

Cook Time: **50** Minutes

Total Time: **60** Minutes

INGREDIENTS

- 10 cloves garlic
- 2 onion
- ½ lemon
- 2 beets
- 3 carrots
- 1/3 tsp turmeric
- 1/3 tsp oregano
- 1 ½ cup vegetable broth
- 1/3 tsp black pepper
- 2 cups broccoli
- 3 bay leaves
- 1/3 tsp salt

DIRECTIONS

1. Peel and dice the vegetables
2. Place in a pot of water and bring to a boil
3. Simmer on low for at least 50 minutes
4. Season and serve hot

PARSNIP SOUP

Serves: *8*

Prep Time: *10* Minutes

Cook Time: *50* Minutes

Total Time: *60* Minutes

INGREDIENTS

- 2 cups vegetable broth
- 2 bay leaves
- 1 tsp salt
- 2 lbs parsnip
- 1/3 cup olive oil
- 1/3 tsp black pepper
- 1 onion
- 1 stalk celery

DIRECTIONS

1. Scrub and cut the parsnip as you desire
2. Place on a baking sheet and toss with oil, salt and pepper
3. Roast until golden

4. Cook the onion and the celery in hot oil for about 5 minutes then season
5. Pour the vegetable broth over, add the bay leaves and the parsnip in and bring to a boil
6. Once boiling, simmer for 15 minutes
7. Remove the bay leaves and puree the soup using a blender
8. Season and serve

ASPARAGUS SOUP

Serves: **6**

Prep Time: **5** Minutes

Cook Time: **25** Minutes

Total Time: **30** Minutes

INGREDIENTS

- 2 leeks
- 1 onion
- 5 tbs flour
- 2 potatoes
- 1/3 tsp nutmeg
- 2 lb asparagus
- 5 cups vegetable stock
- 1 ½ stalk celery
- Salt
- Pepper

DIRECTIONS

1. Cut the asparagus tips off, and set aside, chopped while cutting the asparagus stalks into desired size pieces

2. Simmer the leeks, potatoes, celery, asparagus and onions in vegetable stock for 15 minutes, covered
3. Add the flour and process the soup using a blender
4. Add the remaining vegetable stock, season and simmer covered for 5 minutes
5. Serve immediately

ONION SOUP

Serves: **4**

Prep Time: **10** Minutes

Cook Time: **50** Minutes

Total Time: **60** Minutes

INGREDIENTS

- 3 cups vegetable stock
- 2 tbs butter
- 4 onions
- 2 cloves garlic
- 4 slices sourdough
- 2 glasses of white wine
- Thyme
- Salt

DIRECTIONS

1. Peel the onions and slice it thinly
2. Cook the onions in melted butter for a few minutes, then add the garlic, thyme, salt and pepper
3. Cook for another 10 minutes

4. Pour the vegetable stock over and allow to simmer covered for at least 40 minutes
5. Add the wine and continue simmering for another 10 minutes
6. Ladle the soup into bowls and cover with the sourdough bread slices
7. Grill for 5 minutes in the preheated grill at 350F
8. Serve immediately

ZUCCHINI SOUP

Serves: 2

Prep Time: 5 Minutes

Cook Time: 20 Minutes

Total Time: 25 Minutes

INGREDIENTS

- 1/3 cup red cabbage
- 1 lemon
- 1 onion
- 2 zucchinis
- 1 head broccoli
- 2 ½ cups vegetable stock
- Parsley

DIRECTIONS

1. Peel and chop the onions
2. Fry in olive oil with broccoli and zucchini until soft
3. Add the vegetable stock and allow to simmer for at least 15 minutes on low
4. Blend half of the soup with parsley then return to pot

5. Serve topped with shredded cabbage and a squeeze of lemon

TURKEY BURGERS

Serves: **4**

Prep Time: **10** Minutes

Cook Time: **10** Minutes

Total Time: **20** Minutes

INGREDIENTS

- 12 oz ground turkey
- 2 cup tomatoes
- 1/3 cup onion
- 5 oz cranberry sauce
- 4 buns
- 1/3 tsp coriander
- 2 cups lettuce
- 1/3 tsp salt
- 2 apples
- ½ tsp black pepper

DIRECTIONS

1. Mix the turkey, chopped apples, coriander, salt, pepper, and cranberry sauce together

2. Form patties from the mixture and place on preheated grill
3. Cook covered for about 10 minutes
4. Place the patty on the lower half of the bun and top with the vegetables
5. Serve immediately

ROASTED SALMON

Serves: 2
Prep Time: 20 Minutes
Cook Time: 60 Minutes
Total Time: 80 Minutes

INGREDIENTS

- 1/3 tsp cinnamon
- 4 salmon fillets
- 2 ½ tbs lemon juice
- 1 tsp cumin
- 1/3 tsp salt
- 3 tsp lemon zest
- ¼ cup pineapple juice

DIRECTIONS

1. Mix the lemon and pineapple juices together in a bowl
2. Place the salmon fillet into the bowl and refrigerate covered for at least 1 hour to marinate
3. Mix the seasonings together and rub over the fish
4. Grill in the preheated grill for about 10 minutes

LUNCH NOODLES

Serves: **4**

Prep Time: **10** Minutes

Cook Time: **20** Minutes

Total Time: **30** Minutes

INGREDIENTS

Noodles:
- 14 oz soba
- 1 ½ green onion
- 1 ½ tsp wasabi paste

Sauce:
- 1/3 cup soy sauce
- 1/3 cup mirin
- 1 1/3 cup dashi broth

DIRECTIONS

1. Heat the mirin in a saucepan then add the dashi stock and soy sauce and bring to a boil
2. Remove from heat and allow to cool
3. Cook the noodles until tender in boiling water
4. Divide the soba into 4 bowls
5. Pour sauce over all bowls

CAULIFLOWER WINGS

Serves: **4**

Prep Time: **5** Minutes

Cook Time: **55** Minutes

Total Time: **60** Minutes

INGREDIENTS
Wings:
- 1 cauliflower head
- 3 tsp onion powder
- 2 tsp cumin
- 1/3 tsp black pepper
- 1 cup flour
- 2 tsp garlic powder
- 1/3 cup water
- 1 ½ tsp paprika
- 1/3 tsp salt
- 1/3 cup almond milk

BBQ Sauce:
- Hot sauce
- 1 ½ tbs butter

Vinegar Sauce:
- 4 tbs vinegar

- 2 tbs water
- 2 tbs butter
- Salt

DIRECTIONS

1. Mix the wings ingredients together
2. Toss each cauliflower floret into the mixture
3. Place the florets onto a lined baking sheet
4. Bake for 15 minutes then flip over and bake for another 10 minutes
5. Prepare each sauce into two separate bowl
6. Toss the baked florets into the sauces and place them back on the baking sheets
7. Bake for another 20 minutes
8. Serve immediately

LETTUCE CHICKEN WRAPS

Serves: **4**

Prep Time: **5** Minutes

Cook Time: **15** Minutes

Total Time: **20** Minutes

INGREDIENTS

- 2 tbs olive oil
- 3 tbs soy sauce
- 2 tbs vinegar
- 1 lb chicken
- 1 heat lettuce
- 3 clves garlic
- 1/3 onion
- 1/3 cup hoisin sauce
- 2 tbs ginger
- 1 ½ tsp Sriracha
- 8 oz water chestnuts
- 2 green onions
- 3 carrots
- Salt
- Pepper

DIRECTIONS

1. Cook the ground chicken in hot olive oil for about 5 minutes
2. Add the onion, garlic, soy sauce, hoisin sauce, ginger, vinegar and Sriracha and cook for another 2 minutes
3. Stir in the green onions and water chestnuts and cook for another 2 minutes
4. Season with salt and pepper
5. Serve the mixture on top of the lettuce leaves

DINNER

EASY OYSTERS

Serves: **8**

Prep Time: **40** Minutes

Cook Time: **40** Minutes

Total Time: **80** Minutes

INGREDIENTS

- 4 dozen oysters
- 1 tsp Tabasco sauce
- 1 rib celery
- 1 bunch parsley
- 1 ½ cups bread crumbs
- 4 tbs Worcestershire sauce
- 1 lb butter
- 2 cups green onions
- 1 tsp Pernod
- Rock salt

DIRECTIONS

1. Saute the celery, onions and parsley in the melted butter for 5 minutes, then add the Tabasco and Worcestershire sauce
2. Reduce the heat and cook for 10 minutes, then add the Pernod and bread crumbs and cook for 5 more minutes
3. Refrigerate for at least 1 hour
4. Shuck and drain the oysters
5. Place the shells on rock salt and place 1 oyster in each shell
6. Blend the refrigerated mixture using an electric mixer
7. Put a tablespoon of mixture onto each oyster
8. Bake for at least 5 minutes at 370F
9. Serve hot

DINNER CHILI

Serves: **8**

Prep Time: **10** Minutes

Cook Time: **8** Hours

Total Time: **8** Hours

INGREDIENTS

- 2 tbs olive oil
- 2 cups chicken broth
- 2 green bell peppers
- 1 can black beans
- 1 can kidney beans
- 3 tsp chili powder
- 2 lbs ground turkey
- 1 red onion
- 3 cloves garlic
- 3 tbs tomato paste
- 28 oz chopped tomatoes
- 2 tsp cumin
- 3 tsp oregano
- Salt
- Black pepper

DIRECTIONS

1. Cook the pepper and onion in hot olive oil for about 4 minutes
2. Add the ground turkey and cook until golden
3. Season and add the tomato paste and garlic, then cook for 2 more minutes
4. Transfer to a slow cooker and add the black beans, tomatoes, chicken broth, kidney beans, cumin, oregano, and chilli powder
5. Cook on low for at least 8 hours
6. Serve topped with cheese

GINGER SALMON

Serves: **4**

Prep Time: **20** Minutes

Cook Time: **10** Minutes

Total Time: **30** Minutes

INGREDIENTS

- 2 tbs honey
- 2 lbs salmon fillets
- ½ cup soy sauce
- 3 tbs orange juice
- 2 tbs ginger

DIRECTIONS

1. Mix the honey, ginger, orange juice and soy sauce together
2. Place the salmon in the sauce refrigerate covered for at least 15 minutes to marinate
3. Place the salmon on a lined pan and broil in a preheated broil for 5 minutes
4. Pour some of the remaining marinade sauce over and broil for 1 more minute
5. Serve with desired side dishes

PORK TACOS

Serves: **4**
Prep Time: **10** Minutes
Cook Time: **30** Minutes
Total Time: **40** Minutes

INGREDIENTS

- 12 tortillas
- 3 tsp cilantro
- 2 lbs ground pork
- 3 tbs olive oil
- 1 cup cucumber
- 5 radishes
- 4 scallions
- 1 cup red cabbage
- 3 tsp garlic powder
- 3 tbs sesame oil
- 3 tbs soy sauce
- 1/3 cup vinegar
- 3 tsp sugar
- 3 tsp Sriracha
- 1 cup sour cream

- Salt
- Pepper

DIRECTIONS

1. Mix the radishes, cucumbers, 2 tsp sugar, vinegar, salt, and pepper together
2. Cook the cabbage and scallions in hot oil until softened
3. Add pork, garlic powder and 1 tsp sugar and cook for another 5 minutes
4. Add the soy sauce, Sriracha, sesame oil and stir, then season with salt and pepper
5. Heat the tortillas and spread sour cream on each, then add the pork mixture and the remaining ingredients
6. Serve immediately

VEGETABLE STEW

Serves: *4*

Prep Time: *10* Minutes

Cook Time: *30* Minutes

Total Time: *40* Minutes

INGREDIENTS

- 2 tsp salt
- 8 oz tomato paste
- 1 eggplant
- 3 tomatoes
- 2 onions
- 2 tsp cumin powder
- Cayenne pepper

DIRECTIONS

1. Dice the eggplant, onions and tomatoes
2. Pour the tomato paste, salt, cayenne pepper, cumin and 1 cup water in a skillet
3. Add the vegetables and bring to a boil
4. Reduce the heat to a simmer and cook covered for at least 20 minutes

STUFFED SWEET POTATOES

Serves: **4**

Prep Time: **10** Minutes

Cook Time: **20** Minutes

Total Time: **30** Minutes

INGREDIENTS

- 2 lbs sweet potatoes
- 1 avocado
- 1/3 cup cilantro
- 1 jalapeno
- 2 tbs olive oil
- 1 cup black beans
- 1 red onion
- 2 garlic cloves
- 1 cup corn
- 1 cup tomatoes
- 2 tbs taco seasoning
- ½ tsp salt

DIRECTIONS

1. Cook the sweet potatoes as you desire
2. Saute the jalapeno and red onion in olive oil for 3 minutes
3. Add minced garlic and cook for 1 more minute
4. Add the black beans, corn, seasoning, salt, and pepper and cook 5 more minutes
5. Scoop out the potato insides and fill with the mixture
6. Serve with sour cream

CHICKEN AND RICE

Serves: **4**

Prep Time: **10** Minutes

Cook Time: **20** Minutes

Total Time: **30** Minutes

INGREDIENTS

- 1 cup rice
- 3 tsp seasoning
- 4 chicken breasts
- 2 ½ tbs butter
- 2 ½ cup chicken broth
- 1 lemon
- Salt
- Pepper

DIRECTIONS

1. Season the chicken with salt, pepper and seasoning
2. Cook in melted butter until golden on both sides
3. Add in chicken broth, rice, lemon juice and remaining seasoning
4. Cook covered for at least 20 minutes

LIVER AND MASHED VEGETABLES

Serves: **4**

Prep Time: **20** Minutes

Cook Time: **40** Minutes

Total Time: **60** Minutes

INGREDIENTS

- 3 tsp rapeseed oil
- 350g sweet potato
- 150g parsnip
- 320g green beans
- 350g swede
- 3 cloves garlic
- 15 g flour
- 4 onions
- 1 pack liver
- 1 cube lamb stock
- Black pepper

DIRECTIONS

1. Cook the onions in hot oil for about 20 minutes

2. Coat the liver with flour and pepper and cook in a pan until brown
3. Add the garlic to the onions and stir in 2 tsp of flour
4. Dissolve the stock cube in 450 ml water, then pour over the onions and bring to a boil
5. Add the liver and cook for 5 more minutes
6. Boil the vegetables covered for about 15 minutes
7. Mash the potato, parsnip and swede together
8. Serve the liver with the mashed vegetables

LEMON CHICKEN

Serves: **4**

Prep Time: **10** Minutes

Cook Time: **20** Minutes

Total Time: **30** Minutes

INGREDIENTS

- 3 tsp garlic
- 5 tbs lemon juice
- 4 tbs butter
- 4 chicken breasts
- ½ cup chicken broth
- 1 ½ tbs honey
- 2 tsp seasoning
- Salt
- Pepper

DIRECTIONS

1. Cook the chicken in melted butter until golden on both sides
2. Mix the lemon juice, chicken broth, garlic, honey, salt, pepper, and seasoning in a bowl

3. Place the chicken on a baking sheet and pour the sauce over
4. Bake in the preheated oven for at least 20 minutes at 350F spooning the sauce over the chicken every 5 minutes
5. Serve with lemon slices

CLASSIC LIVER AND ONION

Serves: **4**

Prep Time: **10** Minutes

Cook Time: **20** Minutes

Total Time: **30** Minutes

INGREDIENTS

- 1 lb liver
- 1/3 cup wine
- 1 onion
- 3 tbs olive oil
- 3 cloves garlic
- Pepper

DIRECTIONS

1. Sauté the onion and garlic in hot oil until tender
2. Add the liver in the center and pour the wine over
3. Cook on low for another 15 minutes turning the liver once
4. Serve seasoned with pepper

DINNER BURGERS

Serves: **4**

Prep Time: **10** Minutes

Cook Time: **20** Minutes

Total Time: **30** Minutes

INGREDIENTS

- 2 tbs oil
- ¾ tsp coriander
- 1/3 tsp cumin
- 1/3 tsp cayenne pepper
- 2 tbs honey
- Hamburger buns
- ¾ tsp paprika
- 1/3 cup tomato sauce
- 1 bell pepper
- 1 onion
- 1/3 tsp salt
- 1 ½ tbs molasses
- Black pepper
- 1 tsp oregano
- 2 tbs Worcestershire sauce

- 1/3 tsp celery seed
- ¾ tsp thyme
- 15 oz tempeh
- 3 cloves garlic

DIRECTIONS

1. Cook the onion in oil for about 5 minutes
2. Cook the tempeh until golden
3. Add the garlic and the pepper and cook for another 3 minutes
4. Add the remaining ingredients and simmer for at least 10 minutes
5. Spoon the mixture on the toasted buns and serve immediately

DINNER NACHOS

Serves: 2
Prep Time: **10** Minutes
Cook Time: **20** Minutes
Total Time: **30** Minutes

INGREDIENTS

- 2 tbs olive oil
- 1 handful cilantro
- Salsa
- Salt
- Pepper
- 1 zucchini
- 10 leaves endive
- 3 tsp garlic
- 8 cherry tomatoes
- 10 mini sweet bell peppers
- Taco seasoning
- 1 onion
- 1 lb turkey
- 1 ½ cup mozzarella
- 1 avocado

- 1 lime

DIRECTIONS

1. Sauté the zucchini, cherry tomatoes, garlic, onion and taco seasoning in a pan
2. Add in the ground meat, season with salt and pepper and cook until no more moisture
3. Prepare the peppers by removing the stem and cutting in half
4. Place them and the endive on a pan and top them with mozzarella
5. Top with the meat mixture and sprinkle the remaining mozzarella
6. Put under the broiler for about 2 minutes
7. Mix the avocado with a squeeze of lemon, salt and pepper
8. Spread on top of the nachos and serve

STUFFED PEPPERS

Serves: **4**

Prep Time: **20** Minutes

Cook Time: **20** Minutes

Total Time: **40** Minutes

INGREDIENTS

- 4 red bell peppers
- ½ cup spinach
- 1 zucchini
- ½ green bell pepper
- 1 onion
- 1 cup mushrooms
- ½ yellow bell pepper
- 15 oz tomatoes
- 1 lb ground turkey
- 3 tbs olive oil
- 2 tbs tomato paste
- 2 tsp Italian seasoning
- 1 tsp garlic powder
- Salt
- Pepper

DIRECTIONS

1. Cut the tops off the peppers, remove the seeds and boil for 5 minutes
2. Cook the turkey in a skillet
3. Remove the turkey and cook in the same skillet the mushrooms, green and yellow pepper, spinach, zucchini and onion until tender
4. Return the meat in the skillet and add in the remaining ingredients
5. Stuff the cooked peppers with the mixture and bake for 15 minutes

PORK TACOS

Serves: **4**

Prep Time: **10** Minutes

Cook Time: **30** Minutes

Total Time: **40** Minutes

INGREDIENTS

- 1 cup cucumber
- 3 tsp sugar
- 3 tsp Sriracha
- 5 radishes
- 1 cup cabbage
- 3 tbs olive oil
- 3 tbs sesame oil
- 3 scallions
- 1 ¾ lbs ground pork
- 12 tortillas
- 3 tsp cilantro
- 3 tsp garlic powder
- 3 tbs soy sauce
- 1/3 cup vinegar
- ¾ cup sour cream

- Salt
- Pepper

DIRECTIONS

1. Mix the cucumbers, vinegar, radishes, 2 tsp sugar, salt, and pepper together in a bowl
2. Cook the scallions and the cabbage until soft
3. Add in the pork meat, the remaining sugar and the garlic powder
4. Heat the tortillas
5. Spread sour cream in the center of the tortilla, top with pork mixture, then add the cucumbers and radishes
6. Serve immediately

FISH TACOS

Serves: **8**

Prep Time: **20** Minutes

Cook Time: **30** Minutes

Total Time: **50** Minutes

INGREDIENTS

- 1 ½ lb fish
- 2 cloves garlic
- 5 tbs olive oil
- 1 ½ tbs chili powder
- 16 tortillas
- Red cabbage
- Cilantro
- 1 lime

Sauce:
- 1 ½ tbs honey
- 1 ½ cup mayonnaise
- 3 tbs cilantro
- 1 lime
- Salt

DIRECTIONS

1. Mix garlic, lime juice, chili powder and 2 tbs oil and place the fish inside
2. Allow to marinate for about 15 minutes
3. Mix the sauce ingredients together using a food processor
4. Heat the tortillas on a hot griddle until golden on both sides
5. Cook the fish in the remaining oil for about 5 minutes
6. Place the ingredients in the center of each tortilla and serve

SMOOTHIES

GREEN SMOOTHIE

Serves: **1**

Prep Time: **5** Minutes

Cook Time: **5** Minutes

Total Time: **10** Minutes

INGREDIENTS

- 1 banana
- 1 nub turmeric
- 1 cup almond milk
- 1 carrot
- 1 green apple
- ½ lemon juice
- 1 handful spinach
- 1 tbs parsley

DIRECTIONS

1. Place all of the ingredients together in a blender
2. Pulse until smooth
3. Serve immediately

CLEANSE SMOOTHIE

Serves: **1**

Prep Time: **5** Minutes

Cook Time: **5** Minutes

Total Time: **10** Minutes

INGREDIENTS

- 2 carrots
- 1 lemon - juice
- 1 ½ apple
- water
- 1 beet
- ½ cup kale steamed
- 1/3 ginger root

DIRECTIONS

1. Place all of the ingredients together in a blender
2. Pulse until smooth
3. Serve immediately

DETOX SMOOTHIE

Serves: **1**

Prep Time: **5** Minutes

Cook Time: **5** Minutes

Total Time: **10** Minutes

INGREDIENTS

- 1 inch turmeric
- 1 cup cherries
- 1 cup spinach leaves
- 1 cup almond milk
- 1/3 cup beets
- 1 apple
- 1 ½ tbs chia seeds

DIRECTIONS

1. Place all of the ingredients together in a blender
2. Pulse until smooth
3. Serve immediately

ZUCCHINI AND AVOCADO SMOOTHIE

Serves: **1**

Prep Time: **5** Minutes

Cook Time: **5** Minutes

Total Time: **10** Minutes

INGREDIENTS

- 1 apple
- 1/3 lemon – juice
- 2 tsp chia seeds
- 1 cup mixed greens
- 1 zucchini
- 2 cups coconut water
- 1/3 avocado
- 1/3 cup coriander
- 1/3 tsp turmeric

DIRECTIONS

1. **Place all of the ingredients together in a blender**
2. **Pulse until smooth**
3. **Serve immediately**

TURMERIC SMOOTHIE

Serves: *1*

Prep Time: *5* Minutes

Cook Time: *5* Minutes

Total Time: *10* Minutes

INGREDIENTS

- 1 red apple
- 2 tsp turmeric
- 1 cup coconut water
- 1 orange
- 1/3 cup almond milk
- 2 tsp cinnamon
- 1 cup ice

DIRECTIONS

1. **Place all of the ingredients together in a blender**
2. **Pulse until smooth**
3. **Serve immediately**

PUMPKIN SPICE SMOOTHIE

Serves: **1**

Prep Time: **5** Minutes

Cook Time: **5** Minutes

Total Time: **10** Minutes

INGREDIENTS

- 1 cup almond milk
- 1 banana
- 1 ½ tbs honey
- ½ tsp cinnamon
- 1 tsp ginger
- ½ cup pumpkin
- 1 pinch nutmeg
- 1 pinch cloves
- Ice

DIRECTIONS

1. Place all of the ingredients together in a blender
2. Pulse until smooth
3. Serve immediately

CARROT SMOOTHIE

Serves: *1*

Prep Time: *5* Minutes

Cook Time: *5* Minutes

Total Time: *10* Minutes

INGREDIENTS

- 10 carrots
- 2 oranges
- 1 beet
- 1 ½ lemon
- 1-inch ginger

DIRECTIONS

1. Place all of the ingredients together in a blender
2. Pulse until smooth
3. Serve immediately

EASY SMOOTHIE

Serves: **1**

Prep Time: **5** Minutes

Cook Time: **5** Minutes

Total Time: **10** Minutes

INGREDIENTS

- 1 cucumber
- 1 handful dandelion greens
- 2 apples
- 1 lemon
- 1 beet

DIRECTIONS

1. **Place all of the ingredients together in a blender**
2. **Pulse until smooth**
3. **Serve immediately**

BEET SMOOTHIE

Serves: *1*
Prep Time: *5* Minutes
Cook Time: *5* Minutes
Total Time: *10* Minutes

INGREDIENTS

- 1 apple
- 5 strawberries
- 1 beet
- 1 mandarin orange
- 1 cup water

DIRECTIONS

1. Place all of the ingredients together in a blender
2. Pulse until smooth
3. Serve immediately

ORANGE SMOOTHIE

Serves: *1*

Prep Time: *5* Minutes

Cook Time: *5* Minutes

Total Time: *10* Minutes

INGREDIENTS

- 2 tbs olive oil
- 3 cups orange juice
- 3 cloves garlic
- ¼ inch ginger
- 1 pinch cayenne pepper
- 1/3 cup lemon juice

DIRECTIONS

1. **Place all of the ingredients together in a blender**
2. **Pulse until smooth**
3. **Serve immediately**

DESSERTS

CHIA PUDDING

Serves: **3**

Prep Time: **10** Minutes

Cook Time: **10** Minutes

Total Time: **20** Minutes

INGREDIENTS

- 6 tbs chia seeds
- 2 tsp vanilla
- 1 cup strawberries
- 1 beet
- 1 tbs maple syrup
- 2 cups almond milk

DIRECTIONS

1. Place the chopped beet, almond milk, vanilla, maple syrup and strawberries in a blender and pulse until smooth
2. Add chia and stir every 5 minutes for 15 minutes
3. Refrigerate for at least 2 hours
4. Serve topped with desired fruits

CHOCOLATE FUDGE PIE

Serves: **8**

Prep Time: **5** Minutes

Cook Time: **10** Minutes

Total Time: **15** Minutes

INGREDIENTS

- ¼ tsp salt
- 10 oz chocolate chips
- 2 tsp vanilla
- 12 oz tofu
- 2 tsp cocoa powder
- 3 tbs milk

DIRECTIONS

1. **Melt the chocolate**
2. **Put everything into a blender and pulse until smooth**
3. **Pour into a pie crust and refrigerate until firm**
4. **Serve cold**

PEACH PARFAIT

Serves: **2**

Prep Time: **10** Minutes

Cook Time: **10** Minutes

Total Time: **20** Minutes

INGREDIENTS
Oatmeal:
- ½ cup oat bran
- 5 drops stevia
- 1 tsp vanilla
- 1/3 cup Greek yogurt
- 1 ½ cup almond milk
- ½ cup rolled oats
- ¼ tsp salt
- 1 tsp cinnamon
- 3 tsp maple syrup

Peaches:
- 2 peaches
- 2 tsp maple syrup
- 2 tbs oil
- 1 tsp cinnamon

- 1 pinch salt

DIRECTIONS

1. Mix the oatmeal ingredients together and refrigerate overnight
2. Sauté the diced peaches in hot oil along with cinnamon, salt and maple syrup for at least 5 minutes
3. Spoon the oatmeal in a glass, top with peaches and top again with oatmeal
4. Serve

BANANA PUDDING

Serves: **6**

Prep Time: **10** Minutes

Cook Time: **20** Minutes

Total Time: **30** Minutes

INGREDIENTS

- 10 almonds
- 1 cup milk
- 1 tsp vanilla
- 4 tbs coconut sugar
- 1 egg yolk
- 2 bananas
- 2 tbs cornstarch
- Sea salt

DIRECTIONS

1. Roast the almonds in the preheated oven for at least 10 minutes at 325F
2. Allow to cool then mince
3. Mix the cornstarch, sugar and salt together in a saucepan

4. Add the egg yolk and mix, then slowly stir in the milk
5. Cook on medium heat until it reaches a pudding like consistency
6. Remove from heat and stir in the vanilla
7. Pour into dessert glasses alternating with banana slices
8. Serve topped with whipped cream

EASY BLONDIES

Serves: **9**

Prep Time: **20** Minutes

Cook Time: **20** Minutes

Total Time: **40** Minutes

INGREDIENTS

- 2 cups flour
- 1/3 cup almond milk
- ½ cup almond butter
- 3 tbs coconut oil
- 2 tsp baking powder
- 10 medjool dates
- 2 tsp vanilla
- 2 flax eggs

DIRECTIONS

1. Mix the dry ingredients together in a bowl
2. Grind up the dates using a food processor
3. Add the almond butter and coconut oil and pulse together

4. Transfer to a bowl and add in the milk, eggs, and vanilla
5. Add the dry ingredients over and mix until well combined
6. Spread the dough into a baking dish
7. Bake for about 20 minutes
8. Serve cold

DATE BALLS

Serves: **24**

Prep Time: **5** Minutes

Cook Time: **10** Minutes

Total Time: **15** Minutes

INGREDIENTS

- 2 tsp vanilla
- 1 cup coconut
- 2 cups medjool dates
- 2 cups walnuts
- 1/3 tsp salt

DIRECTIONS

1. Place the walnuts and coconut into a food processor and pulse until crumbly
2. Add dates, vanilla and salt and process again
3. Form balls from the dough
4. Refrigerate for at least 1 hour
5. Serve

NUTELLA

Serves: *12*

Prep Time: *5* Minutes

Cook Time: *5* Minutes

Total Time: *10* Minutes

INGREDIENTS

- 200g tofu
- 4 tbs cocoa powder
- 2 cups pitted dates
- 2 tsp vanilla
- 1 pinch salt
- 1 cup hazelnuts

DIRECTIONS

1. Peel and toast the hazelnuts
2. Pulse the hazelnuts and the salt using a food processor
3. When buttery, add in the remaining ingredients and blend until a smooth paste is formed

APPLE CRUMBLE

Serves: **6**

Prep Time: **20** Minutes

Cook Time: **20** Minutes

Total Time: **40** Minutes

INGREDIENTS
Crumble topping:
- 2 ½ cup walnuts
- 2 Medjool dates

Filling:
- 4 apples
- 1 tbs lemon juice

Applesauce:
- 2 apples
- 1 ½ tbs lemon juice
- 1/3 tsp nutmeg
- 5 Medjool dates
- 1/3 tsp cinnamon
- 1/3 cup raisins

DIRECTIONS

1. Pulse the nuts and dates using a food processor for the crumble topping
2. Dice the apples and toss them with the lemon juice
3. Pulse the applesauce ingredients using a food processor
4. Stir the applesauce into the filling bowl
5. Serve topped with the crumble topping

SWEET POTATO CUSTARD

Serves: **4**

Prep Time: **5** Minutes

Cook Time: **5** Minutes

Total Time: **10** Minutes

INGREDIENTS

- 1 sweet potato
- 1/3 tsp nutmeg
- Dash of cloves
- ½ cup almond milk
- 1/3 tsp cinnamon

DIRECTIONS

1. Cook the sweet potato and mash
2. Mix with the rest of the ingredients in a food processor
3. Serve warm

CACAO TRUFFLES

Serves: *12*

Prep Time: *5* Minutes

Cook Time: *5* Minutes

Total Time: *10* Minutes

INGREDIENTS

- 2 tbs coconut oil
- 1 cup almonds
- 1/3 cup coconut nectar
- 1 ½ tsp stevia
- Coconut flakes
- 1 cup cacao powder

DIRECTIONS

1. **Mix well all the ingredients in a bowl**
2. **Form balls from the dough**
3. **Dip into coconut flakes**
4. **Refrigerate overnight and serve**

THANK YOU FOR READING THIS BOOK!

Made in the USA
Coppell, TX
14 August 2021